# Turn That Trauma Into Strength

## Learn how to take advantage of your pain

By 

## Karina C. Burrage

Copyright © 2023 by Karina C. Burrage. All rights reserved. No part of this publication may be reproduced, distributed, or transmitted in any form or by any means, without the prior written permission of the author and publisher, except in the case of brief quotations embodied in critical reviews and certain other noncommercial uses permitted by copyright law.

# TABLE OF CONTENTS

# Introduction
# The Power of Resilience

There are threads of joy and pain woven into the tapestry of our lives. Trauma, being a powerful force, frequently leaves a permanent imprint on our hearts and minds. It can be a dark cloud that hangs over us, casting shadows on our daily lives. But what if I told you that amid this darkness, there is the potential for transformation, power, and resilience beyond measure?

This book is a journey of discovery, a map for navigating the perilous terrain of trauma and emerging not just unscathed but even stronger. It stands as a testament to the human spirit's incredible ability to heal and thrive despite profound wounds.

We will investigate how trauma shapes us, but more importantly, we will investigate the skills, insights, and strategies that can transform pain into power. This is a look at the incredible ability of the human soul to find courage in adversity and develop resilience from the ashes of tragedy.

As you turn the pages that follow, remember that you have the ability to rise, heal, and transform. The road may be difficult, but it leads to self-discovery, growth, and, eventually, triumph. So, let us begin our investigation of transforming tragedy into strength because doing so embraces the true potential of resilience.

# Chapter One
# Why Can Trauma Be a Catalyst?

**Awakening Resilience**: Trauma frequently forces people to confront their inner strength and resilience. It forces people to find ways to survive and exist in the face of hardship, demonstrating their ability to overcome adversity.

**Reevaluation of Priorities**: Trauma can change a person's perspective on life, forcing them to reevaluate their priorities and what is truly essential. This can result in a more focused and purposeful life.

**Increased Empathy**: Trauma can make people more empathic and compassionate toward others who are suffering. It might inspire people to help and support others who are in similar situations.

**Post-Traumatic Growth**: Many people go through post-traumatic growth, which is a positive psychological shift that can happen after a stressful event. It is typically associated with a greater appreciation for life, healthier relationships, and a greater sense of personal strength. Trauma can serve as a catalyst for people to make positive adjustments in their lives. It can lead to positive decisions like seeking therapy, improving relationships, or exploring new opportunities.

**Resilience and Adaptability**: Being exposed to and surviving adversity can boost resilience and adaptability. It teaches people how to overcome adversity and develop effective coping skills that may be used for a variety of life difficulties.

**Personal Transformation**: Trauma can be a watershed moment in a person's life, ushering them down a path of self-discovery and personal development. It can lead to a stronger sense of self, a better understanding of one's values, and a commitment to living a more fulfilling life.

While trauma is undeniably painful and difficult, it has the potential to be a catalyst for significant human development and positive change. It serves as a reminder of the human capacity to persevere, adapt, and finally thrive in the face of adversity.

# Chapter Two

# Understanding trauma

Understanding trauma is an important step in transforming it into strength. Trauma is a complex and profoundly personal experience, and understanding its many elements is essential.

## Important aspects to consider when learning about trauma

**Types of Traumas**: Trauma can appear in a variety of ways, including physical trauma (as a result of accidents or injuries), emotional trauma (as a result of emotional abuse or loss), and psychological trauma (as a result of experiences such as combat or natural disasters). It is critical for optimal healing to identify the type of trauma. Trauma has a tremendous impact on both the brain and the body. It can cause the stress response system to malfunction and changes in brain chemistry, resulting in symptoms such as anxiety, depression, and hypervigilance.

**Triggers**: Different stimuli, such as noises, images, or situations that reflect the traumatic experience, might cause trauma. Understanding these triggers is essential for trauma management and rehabilitation.

**Repression and Flashbacks**: As a coping strategy, some people may repress painful memories, while others may have flashbacks or intrusive thoughts. These techniques can differ from one person to the next.

**Complex Trauma**: Some people suffer from complex trauma, which is caused by repeated or prolonged painful experiences, most often in interpersonal relationships. Because of the cumulative impact, it may be very difficult to manage.

**Healing Modalities**: A variety of therapeutic modalities can assist people in addressing and healing from trauma. Conversation therapy, cognitive-behavioral therapy,

EMDR (Eye Movement Desensitization and Reprocessing), and other treatments are available. The type of therapy chosen may be determined by the nature of the trauma as well as individual preferences.

**Resilience and coping strategies**: People often develop coping strategies to cope with the effects of trauma. Recognizing these techniques and their impact on one's life is a necessary step in understanding trauma.

**Support Systems**: A strong support system is essential for trauma healing. Friends, family, support groups, and mental health professionals can all help in the recovery process.

**Self-Care and Self-Compassion**: Activities such as mindfulness, meditation, and physical well-being, as well as self-compassion, can be beneficial in coping with and recovering from trauma. Developing self-compassion is also important for combating negative self-perceptions that may arise as a result of trauma.

Understanding these trauma components is the first step toward healing and development. It enables people to make educated decisions about the best strategies for their circumstances, ultimately transforming trauma into strength.

**Trauma's emotional and psychological consequences**

Trauma's emotional and psychological ramifications can be severe and long-lasting. Depending on the nature of the traumatic experience and the individual's fortitude, trauma can affect an individual's mental and emotional well-being in a variety of ways. The following are some of the most common emotional and psychological consequences of trauma:

**Post-terrible stress disorder (PTSD)**: PTSD is one of the most well-known psychological consequences of trauma. It can emerge as a result of witnessing a terrible event. Flashbacks, nightmares, severe anxiety, and hypervigilance are some of the symptoms.

**Anxiety and Panic Disorders:** Trauma frequently causes anxiety and can contribute to the development of panic disorders. Acute panic, rapid heartbeat, and a sense of impending doom may occur.

**Depression**: Trauma can cause depression or exacerbate pre-existing depressive symptoms. Common symptoms include feelings of hopelessness, sadness, and disinterest in activities.

**Emotional Numbing**: As a way to cope with overwhelming feelings, some trauma survivors experience emotional numbing. This may result in an emotional detachment or a feeling of being emotionally "flat."

**Dissociation:** Dissociation is a psychological defense mechanism that manifests as a sense of separation from one's body or surroundings. It is a psychological approach to removing oneself from the distressing event.

**Guilt and shame**: Trauma survivors may experience intense guilt or shame, especially if they blame themselves for the event. These feelings can be devastating and damaging to one's self-esteem.

**Changes in self-perception**: Trauma can impact one's self-concept and self-esteem. Negative self-concepts, self-blame, and a loss of self-worth are uncommon.

**Substance Abuse**: Some people turn to drugs or alcohol as a coping mechanism for the mental anguish caused by trauma, which can result in substance use disorders.

**Relationship Difficulties**: Trauma can have an impact on a person's ability to form and maintain healthy relationships. Trust issues, difficulties with emotional intimacy, and communication issues are all common. Symptoms of psychological trauma include headaches, gastrointestinal problems, and prolonged discomfort.

**Intrusive Thoughts**: Trauma survivors frequently experience intrusive thoughts about the traumatic incident, which can be distressing and unpleasant.

It's critical to understand that each person's emotional and psychological response to trauma is unique. Not everyone who experiences trauma develops these symptoms, and the severity of the damage varies substantially. Seeking professional assistance, such as therapy or counseling, is frequently an important step in addressing and resolving these emotional and psychological concerns.

# Chapter Three
# The Healing Path

The trauma healing journey is highly personalized and frequently nonlinear. It consists of several phases and steps that vary from person to person. Here is a synopsis of the healing process:

**Acknowledgment**: Recognizing that you have experienced trauma is the first step in healing. Acceptance might be difficult since it may need recalling terrible memories and feelings.

**Seeking Help**: It is critical to seek help while recovering. Friends, relatives, support groups, or mental health professionals may be able to help. A strong support network is essential for providing emotional validation and guidance.

**Recognizing Trauma**: As previously stated, recognizing the nature of trauma, its repercussions, and how it has affected you is an important part of the recovery process. It could assist you in making sense of your experiences and regaining your sense of self.

**Therapeutic Interventions**: For many people, therapy is an important element of their healing process. Various treatments, including cognitive-behavioral therapy, EMDR, and trauma-focused therapy, can assist patients in processing their experiences and developing coping mechanisms.

**Emotional Expression**: Typically, healing requires the expression of feelings that have been suppressed or avoided. This can be accomplished through writing, art, or talking with a trusted person.

**Building Resilience**: Building resilience and coping skills is an important part of the healing process. This involves learning to deal with triggers and stress, developing healthy strategies to deal with emotional issues, and developing a stronger sense of self.

**Forgiveness and Compassion:** Healing may necessitate forgiving yourself and others. It can be a transformative procedure that aids in the release of emotional burdens associated with trauma.

**Reframing the narrative**: Many people find healing by reframing their personal tales. This requires shifting from a victim mentality to a survivor mentality, as well as recognizing the traits and growth that have emerged from their experiences.

**Self-Care**: Techniques for self-care, such as mindfulness, meditation, physical activity, and a healthy lifestyle, are critical for maintaining emotional and psychological well-being.

**Reconnecting with Life**: Individuals might reconnect with life in meaningful ways as they heal. This may entail mending relationships, pursuing passions, and setting and achieving personal goals.

**Post-Traumatic Growth**: The healing journey can result in post-traumatic growth, which includes a greater appreciation for life, healthier relationships, and a sense of purpose and meaning.

**Ongoing Care**: Healing is a continuous process rather than a one-time event. Individuals may continue on their recovery road and practice self-care practices to maintain their well-being.

## Acceptance of one's history

Accepting your history is a critical step in moving forward after trauma. Here's why it's critical, as well as some tips to aid you along the way:

### Why Is It Necessary to Accept Your Past?

**Healing:** Acceptance is the basis on which healing is built. It allows you to accept the reality of what you've experienced and the impact it's had on your life.

**Reduces Emotional Burden**: Avoiding or denying your history can lead to emotional repression, which is harmful to your mental and emotional well-being. Acceptance allows you to get rid of some of your emotional baggage.

**Encourages Self-Compassion**: Acceptance means treating yourself with respect and understanding, rather than blaming or condemning yourself. It's a way of saying you did your best with the resources and information available at the time.

**Aids in Coping**: Recognizing your past allows you to better understand the causes and obstacles that may arise in the present. This understanding can aid you in developing more effective coping mechanisms.

## Strategies for Accepting Your Past

**Self-Reflection**: Take some time to think about how your previous experiences have shaped you. Writing in a journal or speaking with a trusted friend or therapist might be beneficial.

**Mindfulness**: Mindfulness practices can assist you in remaining present and nonjudgmental when reflecting on your past. It fosters an acceptance and self-compassion attitude.

**Seek Professional Assistance**: A therapist or counselor can help you embrace your history in a safe and supportive environment.

**Forgiveness**: Think about forgiving yourself and others who were engaged in the tragic events. Forgiveness does not imply acceptance of what occurred, but it may release you from the emotional burden associated with guilt and resentment.

**Letting Go**: Acceptance might mean letting go of the desire for things to be different. You can't change what happened in the past, but you can change how you react to it now.

**Self-Care Routines**: Develop self-care routines to promote your physical and emotional well-being. This may provide a sense of familiarity and stability, making embracing your history easier.

**Support Network**: Talk about your feelings and experiences with friends or a support group. Knowing you're not alone may be reassuring.

**Education**: Gain a better understanding of trauma, its effects, and the rehabilitation process. Knowledge can help you along your path to acceptance.

Accepting your past does not mean erasing the pain or memories of trauma; rather, it means admitting their presence in your life and figuring out how to coexist with them while building a brighter and more resilient future. It is a time-consuming, patient, and self-compassionate process, but it is a necessary step toward healing and personal growth.

# Chapter Four
# Building Resilience

Emotional strength is strongly related to resilience, the ability to recover from adversity. Resilience is a talent that may be learned rather than a natural trait. Here's how to develop resilience:

**Coping Strategies**: Identify appropriate coping skills to manage discomfort. Deep breathing techniques, progressive muscular relaxation, or obtaining expert help to build effective coping mechanisms are examples of such techniques.

**Self-Compassion**: Practice self-compassion by treating yourself with the same care and understanding that you would give to a good friend. Be kind to yourself, especially when experiencing difficult emotions.

**Positive Self-Talk**: Refrain from negative self-talk and replace it with positive affirmations. Use affirmations to boost your confidence, such as "I am strong," "I can get through this," and "I deserve to be happy."

**Set Realistic Goals**: Set appropriate goals for your rehabilitation journey. Each small step toward development increases your emotional power and overall resilience.

Emotional strength is the inner fortitude that allows us to confront life's challenges, particularly the aftermath of trauma, with resilience and grace. It is about developing the ability to not only cope with but thrive in the face of adversity. In this chapter, we will address how to develop emotional strength as a vital component of trauma recovery.

# 1. Recognize and Accept Emotions

The first step toward developing emotional strength is recognizing and accepting your emotions. Trauma can unleash a torrent of emotions ranging from rage and horror to sadness and remorse. It is critical to acknowledge and validate these feelings rather than suppressing or rejecting them. Here are some strategies to assist you:

**Mindfulness**: Use mindfulness to become more aware of your emotions as they arise. This can help you analyze your feelings without judgment and keep them from overwhelming you.

**Journaling**: Write in a journal to express your emotions and thoughts. Writing can provide a safe outlet for processing thoughts and gaining insight into your emotional environment.

**Seeking Help**: Share your feelings with trusted friends, family, or a therapist. Opening up to others can provide emotional validation and alleviate the strain of carrying your feelings alone.

## 2. Emotional Regulation

Emotional strength also includes the ability to regulate your emotions. Trauma can result in major emotional reactions, and learning to regulate these feelings is critical. Consider the following tactics:

**Emotion Regulation Techniques**: Learn emotional regulation techniques such as grounding exercises, self-soothing practices, and the ABCD approach (awareness, balance, choice, and discipline).

**Deep breathing exercises**: Deep breathing exercises can help relax the nervous system and reduce emotional reactivity. When you're feeling overwhelmed, try diaphragmatic breathing to help you ground yourself.

**Healthy Outlets:** Find appropriate outlets for your emotions, such as physical activity, artistic activities, or relaxation techniques such as meditation.

Developing emotional strength is a life-changing process that allows you to face hardship and tragedy with courage and grace. It's about identifying, controlling, and nurturing your emotions in a way that promotes healing and growth. Remember that developing emotional strength is an ongoing process, and each step forward is a testament to your inner power and ability to heal.

## Utilizing Self-Compassion

Self-compassion is a powerful and transformative practice that can be especially effective when healing from trauma. It entails treating yourself with the same compassion and understanding that you would extend to a good friend. We will look at the concept of self-compassion and how to use it to heal yourself.

# Importance of Self-Compassion

Self-compassion is essential for a variety of reasons:

**Healing from Trauma**: Trauma frequently results in negative self-perceptions and self-blame. Self-compassion counteracts these harmful ideas by encouraging self-acceptance and self-forgiveness.

**Emotional Resilience**: Self-compassion assists individuals in managing difficult emotions more effectively, reducing the risk of emotional suppression and distress.

**Reducing Self-Criticism**: Trauma survivors frequently engage in self-criticism. Self-compassion enhances self-kindness and lessens the intensity of self-judgment.

**Coping with Triggers**: Self-compassion buffers the emotional impact of trauma triggers, allowing for a more balanced and compassionate reaction.

## Cultivating Self-Compassion

Let's look at ways you can cultivate self-compassion in your life:

**Self-Kindness:** Treat yourself with the same love and understanding that you would show to a good friend. When you make mistakes or experience failures, respond with self-encouragement rather than self-criticism.

**Mindfulness:** is a critical component of self-compassion. Be attentive to your ideas and feelings without passing judgment. Recognize that pain is a part of the human experience and that you are not alone in your sadness.

**Self-Comparison**: Avoid comparing oneself to others, especially in the context of trauma and healing. Remember that everyone's journey is unique, and it's okay to not be where someone else is in their recovery process.

**Self-forgiveness:** Exercise self-forgiveness for any perceived faults or deficiencies. Recognize that you did the best you could with the resources and knowledge available at the time.

**Self-Care**: Put self-care first in your daily routine. Participate in activities that promote your well-being, such as exercise, meditation, or creative outlets. Self-care promotes the belief that you are worthy of love and attention.

**Journal of Self-Compassion**: Consider keeping a self-compassion notebook to record your self-compassionate thoughts and reactions to difficult experiences. Consider your progress in cultivating self-compassion.

**Seek Professional Help**: If self-compassion is difficult for you, or if self-criticism is deeply ingrained in you, seek the help of a therapist or counselor. They can provide strategies and support that are tailored to your specific needs.

## The Role of Self-Compassion in Trauma Recovery

Self-compassion isn't about getting rid of the pain or the memory of trauma; it's about accepting the suffering you've experienced and finding a way to live with it. Self-compassion supports the belief that you are worthy of care, love, and healing, regardless of your past experiences. It provides a path toward self-acceptance and emotional well-being, allowing you to navigate the challenges of trauma recovery with greater resilience and self-kindness.

Remember that cultivating self-compassion is a journey, not a destination. Be patient with yourself, and celebrate each step forward on your path to self-compassion and recovery.

# Chapter Five

# Finding Purpose and Meaning

Trauma has the power to undermine the very roots of our existence, leaving us grappling with grief, perplexity, and a horrible sense of loss. However, even in the midst of adversity, there is the chance of discovering purpose and meaning that can be transformative. In this chapter, we will look at how to find purpose and meaning in life, which is an important step in turning your suffering into strength.

## Quest for Meaning

When a traumatic event occurs, it typically robs life of its significance. Survivors may question the meaning of their suffering. Finding purpose and meaning involves imbuing grief with significance rather than rejecting it. Here's why:

**Resilience:** Purpose and meaning can serve as beacons of hope, providing a sense of direction and a cause to persevere in the face of adversity.

**Post-Traumatic Growth**: The process of seeking meaning can result in post-traumatic growth, a phenomenon in which people emerge from adversity with a greater appreciation for life and a stronger sense of self.

**Emotional Healing**: You can transform unpleasant sentiments into positive motivations by discovering purpose and meaning. It aids in shifting the emphasis from suffering to personal development.

## The Pursuit of Meaning and Purpose

Here are some resources to help you discover meaning and purpose in the aftermath of trauma.

**Begin with self-reflection**: Investigate your core values, beliefs, and interests. What is it that truly important to you? What are your abilities and skills? Consider how your trauma experience has influenced your worldview.

**Establish Personal Objectives**: Set specific, attainable goals that reflect your newfound understanding of what is important to you. These objectives may serve as stepping stones to a more purposeful life.

**Providing Assistance to Others**: Sometimes finding purpose comes from assisting those who have suffered similarly. This can include activism, volunteering, or telling your story to inspire and help others.

**Engage in creative activities**: such as art, writing, or music. These can be wonderful outlets for expressing the breadth of your experiences and discovering new aspects of yourself.

**Rekindle Passions**: Revisit old passions or discover new ones. Engaging in activities that pique your interest may help you rediscover your sense of purpose.

**Seek Professional Guidance:** A therapist or counselor can help you find meaning in your life. They can assist you in exploring your emotions and experiences in a safe and supportive environment.

## The Transformation Technique

Finding purpose and meaning is a process that evolves with time. It is a continuous process that emerges as you grow and heal. It is about understanding that, even in the face of adversity, life can reclaim its richness and significance.

Remember that you are on your own path when you begin this adventure. What gives your life meaning may be different from what gives someone else's life meaning, and that's just fine. Your path is a testament to your fortitude and capacity to prosper in the face of adversity.

### Acceptance of Post-Traumatic Growth

Trauma has the power to devastate our lives and leave us with severe wounds. Nonetheless, there is a remarkable potential for post-traumatic growth within the rubble. We will look at the concept of post-traumatic growth, how it can be used, and how it can turn sorrow into strength.

## The Post-Traumatic Growth Effect

Post-traumatic growth refers to positive psychological changes that might occur as a result of confronting and digesting traumatic events. It's a fundamental change that can result in the following advantages:

**A Greater Awareness of Life's Preciousness and Fragility:** Many trauma survivors emerge with a greater understanding of life's preciousness and fragility. They learn to appreciate the current moment and to be grateful.

**Relationship Strengthening**: Trauma frequently causes a reevaluation of relationships. Survivors can strengthen bonds with loved ones and develop better empathy and understanding.

**Improved Emotional Resilience**: Post-traumatic growth can lead to increased emotional resilience. Survivors have more strength and agility in the face of adversity.

**Personal Strength**: Individuals frequently discover a huge inner strength they were unaware they possessed. This improved power can be put to use in a variety of situations.

**Priorities Reevaluation**: Trauma causes survivors to reconsider their life goals and priorities. It has the potential to lead to more deliberate and meaningful choices.

### Navigating the process of Post-Traumatic Growth

Accepting post-traumatic growth necessitates navigating a process that is both personal and nonlinear. Here's how you can join this life-changing adventure:

**Self-reflection:** Begin by reflecting on your experiences and how trauma has altered you. Consider the challenges and opportunities that have arisen from your journey.

**Look for Help:** Rely on trusted friends, family, or a therapist for help. Talking about your feelings and experiences can be an important part of the growth process.

**Adopt Resilience**: Develop resilience by practicing coping strategies, identifying healthy responses to triggers and difficulties, and acknowledging your ability to overcome adversity.

**Determine your goals**: Create personal goals and desires that reflect your post-traumatic development. These objectives can serve as a road map for your next steps.

**Develop Your Self-Compassion**: Be kind to yourself and work on developing self-compassion. Recognize that you are a survivor who has endured and grown as a result of adversity.

Mindfulness: When thinking about your trauma, practice mindfulness to stay present and non-judgmental. This promotes acceptance and self-compassion.

## The Journey Continues

Post-traumatic growth is a continuing journey, a transformational process that occurs over time. It is not about erasing trauma memories, but about transforming them into sources of strength, resilience, and understanding. You become a testament to the incredible human power to heal, grow, and find courage even in the face of adversity as you travel this path.

# Chapter Six
# Overcoming Challenges

The path from suffering to strength can be filled with difficulties, roadblocks, and hurdles. Overcoming these obstacles is a critical aspect of the journey. In this chapter, we will talk about common roadblocks and strategies for overcoming them.

## Common Obstacles in the Healing Process

**Trauma Triggers Resurfacing**: Trauma triggers can resurface unexpectedly, producing extreme emotional distress and re-traumatization.

**Emotional Turmoil:** Dealing with overwhelming emotions such as fear, fury, and grief can be difficult.

**Self-Doubt:** Self-doubt, self-blame, and negative self-perceptions can all hinder your progress.

**Reluctance to Seek Help**: It can be difficult to get over the stigma associated with mental illness and seek out professional help.

**Isolation from loved ones**: Trauma can cause emotions of isolation and alienation from loved ones.

**Intrusive Thoughts**: Intrusive thoughts about the traumatic occurrence can interfere with your everyday life.

## Strategies for Overcoming Obstacles

**Develop Coping Skills**: Developing coping skills can assist you in dealing with triggers and emotional pain. Techniques such as grounding exercises and self-soothing activities can help.

**Self-Compassion**: Develop self-compassion to combat self-doubt. Give yourself the same compassion and empathy that you would give to a friend.

**Mindfulness**: Use mindfulness to stay present and nonjudgmental when confronted with difficulties. This can help you respond to challenges with greater resilience.

**Seek Professional Help**: If your problems seem insurmountable, don't be afraid to seek help from a therapist or counselor. They can offer strategies and advice tailored to your specific situation.

**Network:** During difficult circumstances, rely on your support network. Friends, family, and support groups can all provide empathy and encouragement.

**Progress Tracking:** Keep a notebook to document your development and reflect on your accomplishments, no matter how minor they may appear.

**Resilience building:** Improve your resilience by practicing coping skills and learning healthy ways to respond to triggers and difficulties. Resilience allows you to recover from adversity.

**Patience and perseverance**: Overcoming issues is a continuous process, not a one-time effort. It necessitates perseverance, patience, and attention to your recovery process. Remember that dealing with and overcoming these challenges demonstrates your inner strength and resilience. Each obstacle you overcome brings you one step closer to transforming tragedy into strength.

## Navigating Triggers

Triggers are unpleasant memories that can cause distressing emotional and physical reactions. Learning to navigate triggers is a vital component of trauma recovery. We will explain how to detect triggers, how to control and minimize their influence.

## Recognizing Triggers

Triggers can take many forms, such as sights, sounds, smells, or events that remind you of the traumatic event. They have the ability to bring back traumatic emotions, memories, and physical sensations. Understanding triggers is critical because it enables you to:

**Reduce Emotional Suffering**: By identifying triggers, you can respond to them in a way that minimizes emotional suffering.

**Improve Emotional Regulation**: Trigger-control strategies can help you regain control of your emotions and reactions.

**Enhanced Quality of Life:** Navigating triggers successfully can lead to an enhanced quality of life by limiting the disruption they can cause.

## Detecting Triggers

**Emotional Reactions**: Pay attention to acute emotional reactions that appear to arise for no apparent reason. These emotions could be linked to triggers.

**Physical Reactions**: Take note of any bodily sensations that occur in response to certain events or stimuli, such as increased heart rate, perspiration, or muscle strain.

**Flashbacks**: Flashbacks are vivid, disturbing memories of the upsetting occurrence. They are frequently associated with triggers and may be a key indicator.

**Situational Intelligence**: Avoid circumstances or places that make you feel uneasy or unsafe, as they may be triggering.

**Dreams and Nightmares**: Pay close attention to the content of your dreams and nightmares because they may give information about your triggers.

## Managing Triggers

Managing triggers is a continuous exercise that might be difficult yet manageable. Here are some suggestions to help you cope:

**Grounding Techniques**: Grounding exercises, such as the 5-4-3-2-1 method, can help you stay in the present moment when you are triggered.

**Breathing Exercises**: Deep breathing exercises can help you relax and regain control of your emotions.

**Self-Soothing**: Self-relaxing techniques include wrapping yourself in a warm blanket, hugging a soothing object, or inhaling calming smells such as lavender.

**Mindfulness:** Mindfulness techniques can help you observe and accept the feelings that are triggered without judgment. This can lessen the emotional impact.

**Seek Professional Help**: If triggers are really disruptive, consider therapy or counseling to develop specialized coping methods.

**Desensitization**: With the help of a therapist, gradual exposure to triggers in a controlled and safe environment can reduce their impact over time.

## Making a Trigger Management Strategy

Creating a trigger management strategy is a proactive approach to dealing with triggers. Detecting triggers, recognizing early warning signs of distress, and developing ways to mitigate their influence are all part of it.

Triggers can be formidable obstacles in the trauma recovery process, but they are not insurmountable. You can regain control of your emotions and gradually reduce their impact on your daily life by recognizing and carefully managing triggers. Remember that this is a journey of learning, self-discovery, and resilience and that you can overcome these obstacles as you work to transform trauma into strength.

# Chapter Seven

# Recovering from Self-Destructive Coping Patterns

Self-destructive coping mechanisms may be one of the most difficult aspects of trauma healing. In this chapter, we will discuss how to recognize these patterns, how they affect your healing journey, and how to break free from them.

## Recognizing Self-Destructive Coping Mechanisms

Substance abuse, self-harm, avoidance, and other self-destructive coping strategies are examples. Finding these patterns is an important first step. Keep an eye out for signs such as:

**Substance Abuse**: Substance Abuse is defined as an excessive dependency on alcohol, drugs, or other substances to numb emotional suffering.

**Self-Harm**: Engaging in self-harming actions as a coping method for emotional suffering.

**Isolation:** Withdrawal from social interactions and support, resulting in feelings of loneliness and despair.

**Dissociation:** The act of disconnecting from one's thoughts, feelings, and surroundings to avoid unpleasant memories or emotions.

**Repetition of Traumatic Events:** Taking part in actions that recreate aspects of the trauma, often as a kind of self-punishment or an attempt to regain control.

### The Consequences of Self-Destructive Coping

Self-destructive coping mechanisms can exacerbate the emotional and psychological consequences of trauma, resulting in a vicious cycle of misery. They can amplify feelings of guilt, humiliation, and despair. Recognizing the toll, they take on your health is the first step toward breaking free from their grip.

## Recovery Strategies

**1. Professional Guidance:** Seek the help of a trauma-informed therapist or counselor. They can give you guidance, strategies, and a secure place to examine and process your self-destructive behaviors.

**2. Substance Abuse Treatment:** If substance abuse is a problem, look for a substance abuse treatment program that will address addiction as well as underlying trauma.

**3. Self-Compassion:** Practice self-compassion by treating oneself with kindness and understanding, especially in difficult situations.

**4. Alternative Coping Strategies:** Work with your therapist to develop healthier coping strategies to replace self-destructive tendencies. Mindfulness, grounding practices, and emotional regulation techniques may be included.

**5. Social Support:** Reestablish contact with your support system. Friends, relatives, and support groups can provide empathy and encouragement.

**6. Goal Setting:** Set small, attainable goals for yourself to feel accomplished and empowered.

**7. Pay Attention to factors:** Be aware of the factors that lead to self-destructive coping. Create measures to lessen and reduce their influence.

**8. Self-Care:** Prioritize self-care and well-being habits to cultivate emotional and mental wellness.

## Breaking Free and Healing

Recovering from self-destructive coping behaviors is a tough process, but it is a necessary step on your healing road. Recognize that failures may occur, but each step toward breaking away from self-destructive coping is a testament to your strength and resilience. You have the potential to heal, grow, and transform your pain into strength, even in the face of these hurdles. Your story is marked not only by the trauma you've endured but also by your extraordinary capacity for recovery and transformation.

# Chapter Eight
# Self-Care and Well-Being

Self-care and well-being are essential components of the journey from trauma to strength. In this chapter, we'll look at the importance of self-care, well-being practices, and ways to prioritize your mental and emotional health while on the road to recovery.

## Importance of Self-Care

Self-care is the process of caring for one's physical, emotional, and mental health. It is useful in trauma rehabilitation since it:

**Reduces tension**: Self-care activities can reduce tension, making it easier to deal with the emotional effects of trauma.

**Promotes Resilience**: Well-being practices help you recover from setbacks by strengthening your emotional resilience.

**Improves Emotional Regulation**: Self-care helps you manage and regulate your emotions by reducing the impact of triggers and upsetting memories.

**Improves Self-Compassion**: Caring for oneself demonstrates self-compassion and self-kindness.

**Self-Care Methods**

1. Physical Self-Care: Regular exercise releases endorphins and reduces stress.

   - Make a healthy diet a priority to nourish both your body and mind.

   - Get enough sleep; relaxation is essential for emotional well-being.

2. Emotional Self-Care: Use mindfulness and meditation to gain emotional control and stay grounded.

   - Do things that make you happy and relax.

   - Seek professional help to deal with emotions and trauma.

3. Social Self-Care: Develop positive relationships with friends and family.

   - Establish boundaries to protect your emotional well-being and healthy relationships.

   - Attend trauma survivors support groups to connect with others who understand your experiences.

4. Creative Self-Care: - Participate in creative activities that promote self-expression and emotional release, such as art, writing, music, or other hobbies.

5. Professional Self-Care: Recognize the need of work-life balance and take necessary pauses.

   - To avoid burnout, set firm boundaries in your professional life.

# Prioritizing Well-Being

Incorporate healthy behaviors into your everyday routine, such as:

**Thankfulness**: Practice thankfulness by focusing on what is good in your life. A thankfulness notebook can be a helpful activity.

**Positive Affirmations**: Use positive affirmations to combat negative self-talk and cultivate self-compassion.

**Relaxation and Mindfulness**: To stay grounded, practice mindfulness exercises, deep breathing methods, or relaxation activities regularly.

**Goal setting:** establishing significant objectives that reflect your values and preferences.

**Seeking Professional Assistance:** Include therapy or counseling in your well-being strategy.

## Making Self-Care Work for You

Practices for self-care and well-being should be tailored to your specific needs and preferences. Try out a few different tactics to determine which ones are most effective for you. Remember that self-care is a must on your journey of healing and progress, not a luxury.

# Conclusion

Self-care and well-being are not selfish behaviors, but rather necessary components of overcoming trauma and translating it into strength. Prioritizing your mental and emotional health lays a solid foundation for your path and equips you to face the challenges of recovery with greater resilience and self-compassion.

## Embracing a More Powerful Self

You've taken a profound and courageous route of healing and growth in your journey to transform trauma into strength. You've dug deep into your emotions, faced adversities, and harnessed the force of resilience along the road. Your narrative exemplifies the incredible human capacity to not only survive but thrive in the face of hardship.

You've come across the following things on your journey:

**The Search for Meaning**: You've learned that even in the darkest of circumstances, life can regain richness and significance by seeking purpose and meaning in your experiences.

**Embracing Post-Traumatic Development**: You've seen the transforming power of post-traumatic growth, and you realize how adversity can lead to greater appreciation, resilience, and personal strength.

**Overcoming Challenges**: Your perseverance and dedication have enabled you to meet and overcome the barriers in your path, diminishing the emotional and psychological impact of trauma.

**Coping Techniques**: Your coping skills have given you the tools you need to deal with upsetting emotions, triggers, and setbacks.

**How to Navigate Triggers**: You've mastered the art of identifying and handling triggers, allowing you to recover control of your emotions and reactions.

**Self-Care and Happiness:** You've fostered your emotional and mental health by emphasizing self-care and well-being, displaying self-compassion and self-kindness.

Remember that your healing is a unique and ongoing process as you continue on this journey. It's about accepting a stronger self, not deleting it, but changing it as a source of empowerment. Each step forward, no matter how tiny, demonstrates your inner strength and capacity to recover. You are characterized by your courage, resilience, and the strength you've discovered within yourself, not by your trauma. Accept this stronger version of yourself since it demonstrates your extraordinary capacity for growth and transformation. Your narrative is one of perseverance, hope, and the enduring strength of the human spirits